LOVE AND LAUGHTER IN FULL BLOOM

BY

RAYMOND C. DOTY

DISCLAIMER

TABLE OF CONTENTS

CHAPTER 1

Unexpected Encounters

Ryan and Beatrice have a chance encounter at a local café, The Brew Haven, renowned for its cozy ambiance and delicious coffee. Ryan, with his disheveled hair and mischievous smile, catches Beatrice's eye as he playfully teases the barista. Intrigued, Beatrice, a bookworm with a penchant for quirky accessories, musters up the courage to strike up a conversation.

Their banter flows effortlessly as they discover shared interests, from their love for classic literature to their mutual appreciation for cheesy romantic comedies. Laughter echoes through the café as they exchange witty remarks and playful comebacks.

Ryan is drawn to Beatrice's intelligent charm, and Beatrice finds Ryan's charisma irresistible. Little do they know that this accidental meeting will be the start of something extraordinary.

CHAPTER 2

Sparks Fly

Fate intervenes once again when Ryan and Beatrice find themselves attending a mutual friend's party. As they step into the vibrant venue, their eyes lock, and an undeniable spark ignites between them. Nervous yet excited, they find themselves gravitating towards each other, seeking solace in the familiar presence they've come to cherish.

The evening unfolds in a whirlwind of shared laughter, stolen glances, and heartfelt conversations. Ryan surprises Beatrice with his thoughtful gestures, like saving her from a boring conversation or making her laugh when she spills her drink. In the midst of the party's chaos, they steal moments of intimacy, connecting on a deeper level. It becomes clear that their connection is not just based on humor but on an inexplicable emotional resonance.

CHAPTER 3

Awkward Beginnings

Emboldened by their electric chemistry, Ryan decides to take the initiative and ask Beatrice out on a proper date. Eager to impress her, he plans a romantic evening at a trendy restaurant known for its delectable cuisine. However, fate has other plans for their romantic rendezvous.

As the evening unfolds, a series of comedic mishaps disrupt their plans. From a spilled glass of wine that stains Beatrice's dress to an embarrassing encounter with a mischievous stray pigeon, their carefully orchestrated evening descends into delightful chaos. Despite the mishaps, their laughter remains infectious, and they find themselves bonding over their ability to embrace the unexpected.

CHAPTER 4

Blossoming Friendship

Undeterred by their initial awkwardness, Ryan and Beatrice continue spending time together, nurturing a deep and genuine friendship. They explore the city's hidden gems, from cozy bookstores to scenic parks, reveling in each other's company.

During their adventures, they discover shared passions, such as their love for karaoke nights and impromptu dance-offs. Their laughter becomes the soundtrack of their blossoming relationship, creating cherished memories and weaving an unbreakable bond between them. They confide in each other, sharing their dreams, fears, and quirky idiosyncrasies.

As the days turn into weeks, Ryan and Beatrice find solace in the comfort of their friendship, even as their feelings begin to evolve into something more profound.

CHAPTER 5

Comedy of Errors

Ryan and Beatrice's journey to love is not without its fair share of comedic mishaps. Miscommunication and misunderstandings seem to follow them wherever they go, adding both frustration and laughter to their growing relationship.

A string of misadventures ensues, including a series of misinterpreted text messages that lead to hilarious misunderstandings. They find themselves accidentally double-booking events, resulting in comical situations where they have to navigate between conflicting commitments.

Despite the chaos, Ryan and Beatrice's connection strengthens as they learn to communicate better and appreciate each other's quirks. They realize that life's absurdities can be the catalyst for deep connections and unforgettable moments. Through their shared laughter and ability to find joy in the most awkward situations, they learn to embrace the unexpected twists and turns of their romance.

One evening, as they plan a surprise date for each other, they both unknowingly decide to recreate a scene from their favorite romantic comedy movie. The result is a hilarious collision of misaligned expectations, mistaken identities, and a chaotic yet endearing rendezvous that leaves them doubled over with laughter.

Their friends also play a role in their comedy of errors, unintentionally adding to the confusion. From well-meaning but misguided matchmaking attempts to accidental eavesdropping on private conversations, their friends become unwitting accomplices in the unfolding comedy of their love story. Throughout the missteps and mishaps, Ryan and Beatrice's bond grows stronger. They realize that it's the shared laughter, the ability to find humor even in the most awkward situations, that makes their connection truly special.

As they navigate the challenges of miscommunication and the comedic twists of fate, Ryan and Beatrice begin to recognize the depth of their feelings for each other. Their friendship blossoms into a love that is grounded in trust, understanding, and a shared sense of humor.

With each passing day, Ryan and Beatrice become each other's confidants, pillars of support, and partners in laughter. They discover that love is not just about grand gestures and perfect moments but about finding someone who brings joy, laughter, and a touch of hilarity to every aspect of life.

CHAPTER 6

Love's Pranks

Ryan and Beatrice's friends, sensing the deep connection between the two, conspire to bring them even closer together. With mischievous grins and secret plans, they orchestrate a series of playful pranks, hoping to ignite a spark and push Ryan and Beatrice past their lingering hesitations.

From carefully timed accidental encounters to amusing surprise gifts, their friends create scenarios that force Ryan and Beatrice to confront their feelings head-on. While the pranks are meant to be lighthearted, they add an extra layer of complexity to Ryan and Beatrice's already tangled relationship.

As the pranks unfold, Ryan and Beatrice find themselves embarking on spontaneous adventures, embracing the unexpected twists and turns that come their way. They learn to trust the journey, knowing that sometimes the most magical moments arise from the most unconventional circumstances.

CHAPTER 7

Mixed Signals

As Ryan and Beatrice tiptoe closer to a romantic relationship, they become entangled in a web of mixed signals.

Both afraid of vulnerability and rejection, they inadvertently send confusing messages, leaving them in a state of perpetual uncertainty.

Their conversations become a dance of subtext and hidden meanings, causing humorous misunderstandings and frustrating near-misses. Their friends, ever the well-intentioned instigators, attempt to play matchmakers but only contribute to the confusion.

Amidst the chaos, Ryan and Beatrice realize they need to confront their fears and communicate openly with each other. They embark on a heartfelt conversation, shedding light on their hopes, insecurities, and desire for clarity. Through honest dialogue and shared vulnerability, they navigate the maze of mixed signals, inching closer to a deeper understanding of their true feelings.

CHAPTER 8

Tangled Hearts

Just as Ryan and Beatrice start to find their footing, an unexpected twist threatens to unravel their delicate connection. An old flame resurfaces

in Ryan's life, sparking insecurities
and doubts within Beatrice. Torn
between her growing affection for
Ryan and the fear of getting hurt, she
must confront her own tangled
emotions.

Ryan, realizing the impact of his past
on their present, takes it upon himself
to assure Beatrice of his commitment
and unwavering affection. He proves
his dedication through gestures both
big and small, reminding her that she
is the one he wants to be with.

Together, they navigate the
complexities of their intertwined
hearts, learning to trust each other and
heal the wounds of the past. Their
journey brings them closer, as they
discover that true love requires

embracing vulnerability and overcoming the obstacles that stand in their way.

CHAPTER 9

Moments of Truth

As Ryan and Beatrice's relationship deepens, they find themselves confronting moments of truth that shape their future together. Through shared experiences and intimate conversations, they unveil their deepest dreams, fears, and desires.

They discover that beneath their playful banter and laughter lies a profound connection, a love that transcends the surface-level attraction. It's a love built on understanding, acceptance, and genuine admiration for each other's strengths and quirks.

With each moment of truth, Ryan and Beatrice peel back the layers of their hearts, cementing their bond and solidifying their commitment to one another. They learn that being vulnerable and sharing their innermost selves is the key to true intimacy.

CHAPTER 10

Love in Full Bloom

After overcoming the hurdles of mixed signals and untangling their emotions, Ryan and Beatrice realize that their love has blossomed into something extraordinary. They no longer shy away from expressing their feelings, and their relationship takes on a new depth and intensity.

In this final chapter, Ryan and Beatrice find themselves on a romantic getaway, surrounded by beautiful gardens in full bloom. As they wander hand in hand through the vibrant landscape, they reflect on their

journey together—the laughter, the pranks, the moments of vulnerability, and the strength they've found in each other.

Surrounded by the beauty of nature, Ryan takes a deep breath and decides it's time to take their relationship to the next level. In a moment of heartfelt sincerity, he kneels down, presenting Beatrice with a ring—a symbol of his unwavering love and devotion. With tears of joy streaming down her face, Beatrice nods in affirmation, accepting his proposal and sealing their love in a promise of forever.

Their friends, who have been eagerly rooting for their relationship from the sidelines, appear from behind the blooming flowers, cheering and clapping. The atmosphere is filled with love and celebration as Ryan and Beatrice embrace, their hearts overflowing with happiness.

In the months that follow, Ryan and Beatrice immerse themselves in wedding preparations. Their shared sense of humor shines through as they plan a ceremony that reflects their unique personalities—a celebration filled with laughter, joy, and a touch of whimsy.

On their wedding day, surrounded by family and friends, Ryan and Beatrice exchange heartfelt vows, promising to be each other's constant source of laughter and support. The ceremony is filled with humorous anecdotes, witty remarks, and spontaneous bursts of laughter, encapsulating their journey together.

As the sun sets and the reception begins, the dance floor becomes a stage for their lighthearted antics and their ability to turn even the simplest moves into a comedic masterpiece. They twirl, spin, and laugh together, creating a vibrant energy that infects everyone around them.

With their love in full bloom, Ryan and Beatrice embark on a lifetime of shared adventures, weaving laughter, love, and the joy of each other's company into the fabric of their lives. They continue to find humor in the mundane, embrace the unexpected, and navigate the challenges with a spirit of laughter and resilience.

Their love story serves as a reminder that true happiness lies not only in finding someone who makes you laugh but also in building a deep connection that weathers the tests of time. Ryan and Beatrice's journey is a testament to the power of love, laughter, and the beauty of a rom-com-worthy happily ever after.

www.ingramcontent.com/pod-product-compliance
Lightning Source LLC
Chambersburg PA
CBHW070236260726
48658CB00006BA/2352